D1741287

All About
INFECTION CONTROL

By Laura Flynn R.N., B.N., M.B.A., In consultation with her nurse educator associates and physicians who assisted in contributing and editing.

Thanks also to the following organizations: Center for Disease Control (www.cdc.gov) Infection Control Guidelines. Canadian Association for Wound Care (CAWC), Wound Ostomy Continence Nurses (WOCN) association, The Agency for Health Care Policy (AHCPR), College of Physicians and Surgeons, best practice guidelines

ISBN No: 978 1 896616 66 7

Infection prevention. Infection control. Stop spread of infection. Infection control guidelines.

The publisher, Mediscript Communications Inc., acknowledges the financial support of the Government of Canada through the Canadian Book Fund for our publishing activities.

www.mediscript.net

Printed in Canada

Book and Front Cover design by:
Brian Adamson, www.AdamsonGraphics.net

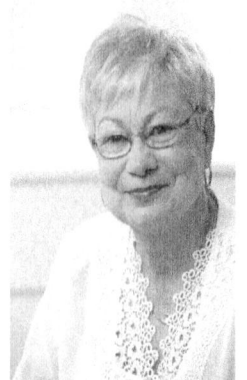

CONTENTS

INTRODUCTION

This book provides basic, non controversial and trusted information that can help a wide spectrum of readers.

The primary objective of the information is to help a person provide effective quality care to a loved one or someone in his or her care.

Reducing the spread of infection is a vital priority and prevention can be as simple as regular and thorough handwashing. This book explains the nature of infection and comprehensively covers all the necessary issues, procedures and tips.

All the information is reliable and was written by a group of eminent nurse educators who ensured the information complies with best practice guidelines and satisfies the various accreditation and regulatory bodies. Because there is so much unreliable information on the internet, you can be assured the "all about" publications are HON (Health On the Net) certified.

This book can be an invaluable aid to:

- A caregiver caring for a relative or friend
- A health worker seeking a reference aid
- A patient or person needing to be transferred
- Any person involved in health care wishing to expand his or her knowledge

---

SOMETHING TO THINK ABOUT...

Life's most persistent and

urgent question is:

What are you doing for others?

Martin Luther King, Jr.

AN IMPORTANT MESSAGE
FROM THE PUBLISHER

Each person's treatment, advice, medical aids, physical therapy and other approaches to health care are unique and highly dependant upon the diagnosis and overall assessment by the medical team.

We emphasize therefore that the information within this book is not a substitute for the advice and treatment from a health care professional.

This book provides generic information concerning how infections begin and how they spread, and the practices you can use to prevent the spread of infections.

With all this in mind, the publishers and authors disclaim any responsibility for any adverse effects resulting directly or indirectly from the suggestions contained within this book or from any misunderstanding of the content on the part of the reader.

Signs that you are over the hill

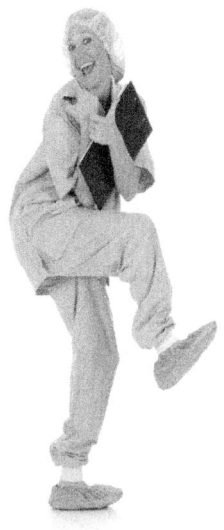

- You run out of breath walking down a flight of stairs

- The speed limit seems excessive

- Your back goes out more often than you do.

- The animals you had as a kid are now extinct.

- At cafetarias, you complain the gelatin is too tough.

HOW MUCH DO YOU KNOW?

This helps to figure out how much you know before you start. In this way you will have an idea as to the gaps in your knowledge prior to reading the content. Please circle to indicate the best answer. Remember, at this stage, you are not expected to know all the answers:

1. The world around us is filled with tiny living things called microorganisms.

a) True

b) False

2. Microorganisms that cause infection are called pathogens.

a) True

b) False

3. Once a pathogen enters a person's body, that person becomes a "portal of exit".

a) True

b) False

4. The best water temperature for handwashing is:

a) Hot

b) Warm

c) Cold

5. A series of events resulting in an infection is called a:

a) Chain of infection

b) Mode of transmission

c) Portal of entry

6. Two ways in which pathogens can be spread are by touch and light.

a) True

b) False

7. It is important to dry your hands well with a paper towel after using an alcohol-based hand cleanser.

a) True

b) False

ANSWERS

1. a) True. Microorganisms are everywhere but we survive them due to our immune system.

2. a) True. Pathogen, from the Greek word "pathos" meaning suffering or emotion, is the term for a harmful microorganism.

3. b) False. When a pathogen enters a person's body, that person is called the "host". "Portal of exit" is explained later in this chapter.

4. b) Warm water is most conducive to cleanliness.

5. a) The chain of infection is explained later in this chapter.

6. b) False. The presence or absence of light will not spread a pathogen.

7. b) False. The alcohol remains active on your hands and will kill any pathogens.

CORE CONTENT
WHAT IS AN INFECTION?

The world around us is filled with tiny living things called **microorganisms.** They are in the air, in water, and in soil. They can be found on objects as well as on people. They also live within animals and humans. These microorganisms are too small to be seen with the naked eye. They can only be viewed through a microscope. See picture below.

Most of these microorganisms are harmless and natural to the body. They can even protect us from getting sick. Each microorganism has a special purpose and is not harmful in its own environment. However, when it invades or enters other areas, it can grow there and cause disease or infection.

For example, Escherichia coli (E. coli) is a common type of bacteria found in our intestines (bowel). It plays an important part in the digestive process (the process of breaking down food substances into forms that can be used by the body). E. coli and other kinds of bacteria are necessary for our bodies to work properly and for us to stay healthy. When E. coli gets into the bladder or bloodstream, however, it can cause infection.

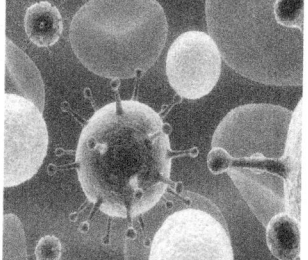

HOW DO MICROORGANISMS GROW?

Microorganisms need 5 things in order to survive and grow. These include:

• **Food.**

Each microorganism needs a different type of food to survive.

• **Water.**

Most microorganisms grow better in moist surroundings.

• **Oxygen.**

Microorganisms require different amounts of oxygen.

• **Temperature.**

Microorganisms need to live within certain temperature ranges. Our body temperature promotes the growth of many microorganisms.

• **Light.**

Microorganisms grow best without light. Sunlight usually kills them or helps to slow down growth.

Microorganisms that cause infections are called pathogens. Bacteria, fungi, and viruses are all pathogens. The common cold is one example of an infection caused by a virus. Pathogens get into our bodies and produce wastes called toxins. These toxins make us sick. Some pathogens cause mild infections while others cause major infections and can do great harm to patients, caregivers, and any other person who may come into contact with them.

WHAT IS THE CHAIN OF INFECTION?

Pathogens may enter the body through different routes (openings) such as breathing passages, eyes, broken skin on the skin, the urinary tract (bladder), and other openings in the body. Once a pathogen has entered a person's body, then that person is called the host. A pathogen can enter your body but not cause an infection.

Six things must be present in order for an infection to occur:

1. Pathogen. The microorganisms (bacteria etc.) that cause the infection

2. Reservoir or source for the pathogen. This is an area where a pathogen can live (usually includes where it can grow). A reservoir can include objects, people, animals, food, insects, soil, or water. The most common reservoir is the human body.

3. Portal of exit. A portal of exit is a route or way for the pathogen to leave the source. The nasal passage or open wounds are two examples of a portal of exit.

4. Mode of transmission. A mode of transmission is a way for the pathogen to be spread. Examples are:

Touch:

Direct contact with a person, animal, or object that has this pathogen. This type of contact most often involves the hands.

Droplet contact:

Can spread to someone within three feet of a person who coughs or sneezes.

Air:

Carried in the air in dust or moisture.

Object:

Carried by an object, food, water or soil.

Animals:

Animals or insects may carry microorganisms from an infected site to a non-infected site.

5. Portal of entry. The way in which a pathogen enters the host. Broken skin areas, the urinary tract, or the breathing passages are examples of portals of entry.

6. Susceptible host. Someone who is at risk for infection. Many people who are elderly and/or ill would be considered susceptible hosts.

This series of events is called the **Chain of Infection** (see Fig. 1). An infection will develop if this chain remains intact. Stop the chain at any point and an infection will not take place.

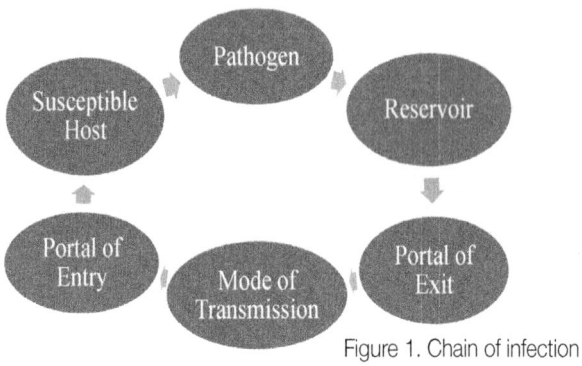

Figure 1. Chain of infection

It is up to you, the caregiver, to work to break this chain so that an infection does not occur. How can you do that? The easiest way is by following proper practices to prevent or control infection.

CONSIDER FOR A MOMENT ...

Think about how pathogens can be carried along each step of the chain of infection from one person to another.

MEDICAL ASEPSIS

Medical asepsis refers to the practices that help to prevent infection. In other words, it involves the things you as a caregiver can do to avoid the growth and spread of pathogens. This is also known as "clean or aseptic technique".

Aseptic techniques will help you keep the people you are caring for and others around you free from infection. Some examples of aseptic techniques include changing someone's bed linen, wearing gloves, and handwashing. Aseptic practices can be used to break each link of the infection control chain. For example:

• To destroy pathogens, regularly cleanse with soap and detergent, disinfect with a number of store-bought disinfectants, or sterilize wound care supplies and other items as needed.

• To reduce or destroy reservoirs, ensure that areas that contain waste or bodily fluids are cleaned or put into their proper containers. This may include items such as bed linens, clothes, tissues, basins, and any other items that may have come into contact with infected material.

- To control the portal of exit, use practices that reduce the chance of pathogens leaving the reservoir. For example, ensure that the person in your care does not have draining wounds that are left open. Clean up saliva and other secretions immediately. Ensure that areas, such as toilets, basin, or utensils, are cleaned regularly.

- To prevent the transmission of pathogens, know how they are spread. Encourage the person to cover his/her mouth while sneezing. You should do the same. All areas that may have come in contact with the pathogen should be kept clean. Soiled items should be cleaned or discarded immediately after use.

- As discussed earlier, harmful microorganisms or pathogens vary in how easily they can be spread or transmitted to people. Assume that all pathogens are easily spread and act to prevent this from happening. Remember that pathogens can attach to your skin and clothing. You can pass them on to other people or objects, or even yourself. For example, when you touch soiled bed linen in someone's bed, pathogens can attach to your hands and uniform. They can then be passed on to another person in your care or transferred to any object in the room.

- To control the portal of entry, try to prevent pathogens from entering the host. Ensure that the person's skin is kept in good condition. Sores or breaks in the skin increase the risk of infection.

- To decrease susceptibility to infection, work with the person to keep him/her as well as can be. Encourage healthy practices such as a balanced diet. Keep items in his/her surroundings clean and free from garbage and clutter to limit exposure to pathogens.

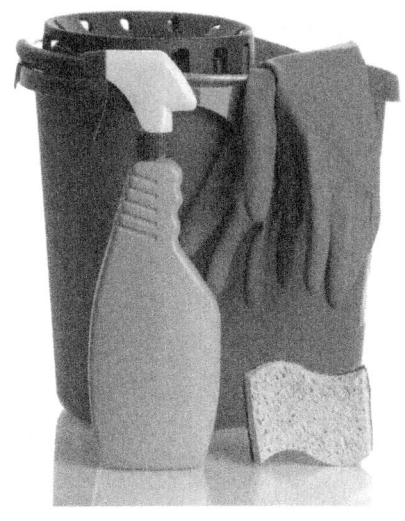

THE DIFFERENCE BETWEEN CLEAN AND DIRTY

One goal of medical asepsis is to separate clean areas from dirty areas to lower the chance of spreading pathogens. For example:

Clean areas

Clean areas have some microorganisms but not the ones that cause infection. Hospitals and nursing homes have a room called a clean utility room. A clean utility room contains clean supplies and a sink. Items that contain pathogens, such as garbage, cannot be carried into the room. Wash your hands before entering this room so you will not carry pathogens in on your hands. A kitchen area or galley in the hospital or home may also be considered a clean room. Waste should not be carried into this room.

Dirty areas

Dirty areas contain things that may carry pathogens. Examples are toilets, soiled equipment, and soiled bed linen. Never carry dirty items into a clean area. For example, when working in someone's home, avoid washing clothes in the kitchen. The kitchen is considered to be a clean area. Soiled clothes and bed linen may contain pathogens. If you bring these items into the kitchen, the pathogens can easily spread to clean surfaces such as countertops, dishes, and appliances.

THE IMPORTANCE OF HANDWASHING

The simple task of handwashing is a practice that is considered vital in all instances of infection control. According the Handbook of Nursing Procedures, handwashing is "the single most important procedure for preventing infection." In order to be effective in controlling infection, handwashing must be done often and it must be done well.

As a caregiver, a major part of your work involves contact or touching the people in your care. This means that you will also come into contact with a number of pathogens. These are easily picked up on your hands when you touch people or objects around them. This is the most common way pathogens are spread. For example, if you wash someone's face, you may touch fluids from the eyes, mouth or nose. These fluids may contain pathogens. These organisms may then be spread to other people, yourself, or objects around you.

Handwashing is the number one way to reduce the spread of disease-causing microorganisms. Most pathogens can be easily removed from your hands using plain soap and water. The importance of handwashing should not be taken lightly. It should never be avoided to save time no matter how busy you become. Many shortcuts are required in the art of nursing to help the nurse and or caregiver survive the day but failing to practice correct handwashing techniques shouldn't be one of them. All caregivers must remember the necessity of washing their hands.

Remember:

Handwashing is the best way to protect you and those around you from infection.

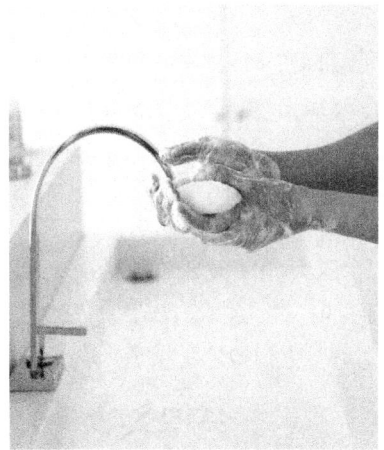

WHEN SHOULD YOU WASH YOUR HANDS?

As a caregiver, you need to know when and how often you should wash your hands. Whether or not handwashing should occur depends on several factors, such as:

- The type of activity. Does it involve touching soiled items or pathogens? For example, are you giving a bed bath or helping a person with toileting?

- The intensity of the activity. Is there a high degree of contact with soiled items or pathogens? For example, are you cleaning someone who has lost bowel control, or who is vomiting or bleeding?

- The length of the activity. Will there be contact with the person and pathogens over a long period of time?

- The series of activities. In what order are you carrying out your tasks? For example, are you changing a soiled bed before you serve someone a meal?

Part of your role as a caregiver is to think about these factors when deciding when you should wash your hands. It has been recommended that caregivers wash their hands:

- When they are obviously soiled

- Before and after contact with the person in their care

- Following contact with a source of microorganisms such as blood, mucus, a broken skin area, or an object that could be contaminated

- Before performing tasks such as giving needles, packing open wounds, or inserting catheters (You may not be required to perform such tasks in your job)

- After removing gloves

CONSIDER FOR A MOMENT...

How many times have you washed your hands at work today? Did you wash your hands in each instance as outlined above?

PEOPLE AT RISK

For different reasons, people are sometimes at greater risk (prone) to infection. If the person in your care has a condition that lowers his/her defenses to infection, or if you are caring for a newborn child, then you must be extra careful with handwashing before each physical contact.

Handwashing with regular soap (bar soap, granule soap, or liquid soap) is suggested when dealing with the average person. A caregiver may be required to use a special soap (antimicrobial soap) when dealing with newborns and those who easily catch infections. These soaps remove pathogens from the deep layers of the skin that may not be washed away with regular soap. You should use regular soap unless you are instructed otherwise.

CONSIDER FOR A MOMENT...
Are you currently caring for someone who is at increased risk for infection? If so, why is he or she at increased risk?

WHAT ABOUT GLOVES?

Gloves should be worn in a number of situations to reduce the risk of spread of infection. Gloves should be worn when there is a chance of coming into contact with blood, body

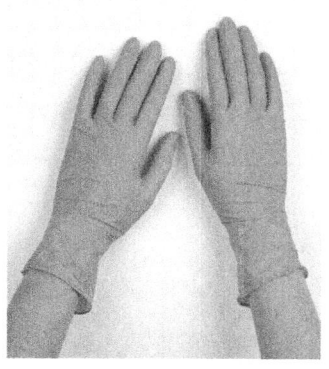

fluids, broken skin, mucous membranes, excretions or secretions (i.e. urine, feces, fluid from open wounds), or contaminated items (those containing a pathogen). One should assume that any person could be infected. Wearing gloves in those situations serves to reduce the chance of transmission of pathogens. Gloves should be taken off immediately after care and thrown away. Don't reuse your gloves.

Workplace policies on infection control, including the use of gloves, may differ somewhat depending on individual needs and federal, state, or local regulations. If these policies are in place where you work, be sure to follow those procedures with respect to infection control and the use of gloves.

Wearing gloves does not mean that you do not need to wash your hands. You should wash your hands even when you wear gloves. Gloves may have small defects or can become torn exposing you to pathogens. Improper fit, prolonged use, prolonged storage, and rings can reduce the barrier protection of gloves. You should wash your hands before you put gloves on and after you take them off.

CASE EXAMPLE

Imagine that you are feeding a confused man in a four-bed room in a nursing home. Another person in the room uses a tissue to wipe the mucus from his nose. You observe as a co-worker, Mary Long, takes the soiled tissue and puts it in the garbage. Although Mary does not know it, the soiled tissue contains pathogens.

Meanwhile, a third person in the room is eighty-six years old and recovering from a serious illness. His name is Mr. Ryan and he requires help with his meal. Without stopping to wash her hands, Mary removes the cover from Mr. Ryan's meal tray, takes the lid off the drinks, and starts to butter the bread.

Using the chain of infection as a guide, discuss how the pathogens may transfer to Mr. Ryan.

Will Mr. Ryan develop an infection as a result of Mary's actions?

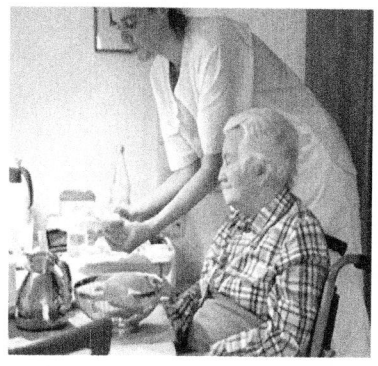

YOUR ANSWERS TO THE CASE EXAMPLE

SUGGESTED ANSWERS TO CASE EXAMPLE

Using the chain of infection as a guide, discuss how the pathogens may transfer to Mr. Ryan.

Pathogens were present in the mucus of the infected person. They exited through that person's nasal passages. By touching infected material on the soiled tissue, Mary may have picked up pathogens on her hands. From there, the pathogens may transfer to the food and dishes of Mr. Ryan. Later, when he touches these items and eats his meal, they may enter through his mouth.

Will Mr. Ryan develop an infection as a result of Mary's actions?

It is impossible to predict with certainty that Mr. Ryan will develop an infection as a result of Mary's actions. From the details in the case, it seems likely that Mr. Ryan was exposed to disease-causing microorganisms. He may also be highly susceptible to disease due to his age and the fact that he is recovering from a serious illness.

On the other hand, however, Mary may not have touched the infected material when she picked up the tissue. Or the light in the room may have quickly destroyed any pathogens that were present. For a variety of reasons, an infection might not occur.

HANDWASHING

PROCEDURES:

Equipment needed

1. Soap. Use bar soap, liquid soap, or soap-filled wipes. Keep bar soap in a holder with drain holes. If bar soap sits in a pool of soapy water, it is considered dirty. The soap holder should be cleaned 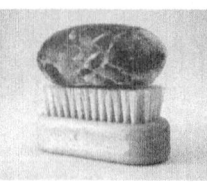 before each new bar of soap is placed in it. If you are using liquid soap or a detergent, the container should be used until it is empty and cleaned before it is refilled.

2. Paper towels. Paper is preferable but clean cloth towels can be used if they are not shared with others.

3. Warm running water. A basin or sink of standing water will not allow for proper cleansing as the pathogens may not be washed away.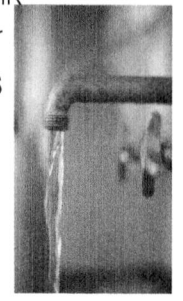

4. Nail brush

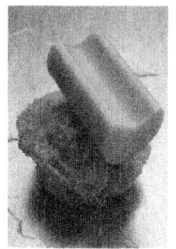

5. Trash container

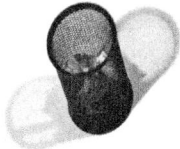

Steps in good handwashing

1. **Keep your fingernails short.** If your nails are not short, they should be trimmed. Long nails can carry a number of pathogens that become trapped underneath and may not be washed away even with proper handwashing. Artificial (fake) nails should not be worn since it has been proven that they carry more pathogens than natural nails.

2. **Remove jewellery from your hands and arms.** This is necessary as microorganisms can grow in the grooves of jewellery and spread to people or objects. A wristwatch with an elastic band may be worn and moved up to the elbow before washing begins. The watch can also be pinned to your clothes.

3. **Check your hands for breaks in the skin.** These can include sores, cuts, or hangnails. You may have to wear gloves to avoid contact with infected substances.

4. **Stand directly in front of the sink.** Your waist should be below the level of the sink. You may have to bend your knees if you are above this level. Do not lean against the sink or get your uniform wet since microorganisms are attracted to moist places.

5. **Use a paper towel to turn on the water.** This will ensure that you do not pick up pathogens from the faucet.

6. **Adjust the water so that it is warm.** Cold water does not produce enough lather from the soap to remove pathogens. Hot water can have a drying effect and be irritating to the skin.

7. **Wet your hands and hold your arms under the running water.** Hold your hands lower than your arms so the water runs from your arms to your hands and fingers into the sink. This prevents pathogens from the hands from getting washed onto the arms. Note: You should always wash from the cleanest area to the dirtiest area.

8. **Apply soap to your hands.** About a teaspoon or 5 ml. is required if you are using liquid soap. If you are using a bar soap, rub it firmly between your hands two or three times before you begin to lather it. Once soap has been applied, wash your hands and fingers. Use plenty of lather and friction for 10 to 15 seconds. Make sure to wash all surfaces of the hand (palm, back, fingers, wrist). Always clean between the fingers as these areas are often neglected and pathogens grow easily there. If your hands are heavily soiled, you may have to wash for longer than 15 seconds.

9. **Make sure lather gets under your nails as well.** Use a nailbrush to scrub under the nails. Add water to the soap so that it does not dry out while you are rubbing.

10. **Rinse your hands with warm running water.** Again, hold your arms downward toward the sink so the water can flow down your arms, over your hands and into the sink.

11. **Use paper towels to dry your hands and arms.** Place them in a garbage or trash container.

12 **Turn off the water using a paper towel to hold the faucet.** This ensures that you do not pick up pathogens from the faucet on your hands.

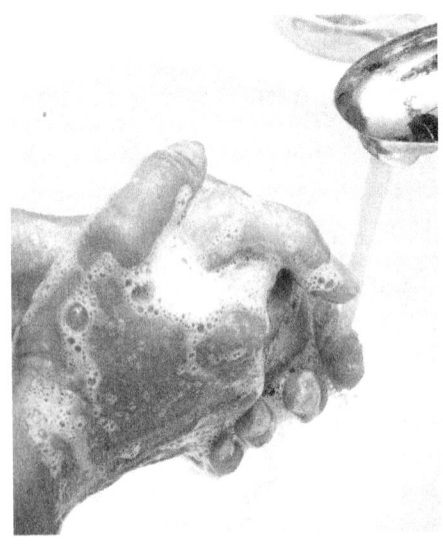

TEACHING THE PERSON IN YOUR CARE

Earlier in this book we discussed the importance of proper handwashing in your work area. Another way to improve infection control is to teach the people in your care how and when to properly wash their hands. The technique that you learn through this book can be demonstrated to them and their families as you talk to them about the importance of not spreading germs.

It is very important that people wash their hands after going to the toilet or commode because they can pick up pathogens on their hands. Handwashing is also important before eating and drinking or when coming in contact with pathogens on tissues, bed linens or wounds.

In your work it is important that you promote handwashing. Be positive and offer help as often as possible. Also be a good role model. The people in your care and their families are more likely to wash their hands when they see you doing it.

HAND CLEANSING GELS

It is well known that caregivers are very busy people and that handwashing is not carried out as often as it should be. This results in high rates of infection and illness. In fact, every year in the United States alone 2 million patients become infected during hospital stays. Many of these infections are life threatening and could be prevented by simple handwashing.

When caring for someone, there may be times when you find it difficult to get your hands washed. This may be because you are very busy or you do not have access to a sink or running water. Whatever the reason, you have learned earlier in this book that you must ensure your hands are clean.

Some workplaces have chosen to use alcohol-based gels in place of handwashing in certain instances. The gels are also called hand sanitizers or hand rubs. They do not require water and are simply rubbed into the hands to kill pathogens. Although they have been used in hospitals in Europe for many years, they are just becoming popular in North America. They can also be found in most pharmacies or stores that sell soaps and other cleansers.

These gels should not replace soap and water. Even though they kill many pathogens, they do not remove dirt and soil. They can be used at times when it is hard to get to a sink.

To use a hand cleansing gel:

- Apply gel so that it covers the hands and fingers.
- Rub into hands briskly for about 30 seconds until the hands are dry.

Note: Towels are not needed as the gel dries very quickly.

The gel is sometimes left at the person's bedside or carried in a pocket for easy access. You should note that, because these gels are alcohol-based, they are flammable. This means they can easily catch fire and should be kept away from areas of high heat or flame.

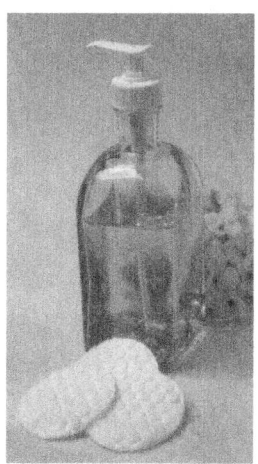

CONCLUSION

The world around us is filled with tiny living organisms. Many of these microorganisms help us to survive. Many others, however, can lead to infections that can cause us great harm. As a caregiver, part of your duty to the person in your care is to know how infections begin and how they are spread.

It is also your responsibility to use practices that prevent the spread of infections. Handwashing is the best way to do this. It is a simple skill that takes only minutes to perform. When carried out on a regular basis, this skill can prevent you and those around you from becoming ill.

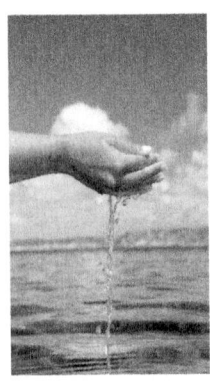

HANDWASHING REMINDERS

DON'T:

• Use a standing basin of water to wash and rinse your hands. Running water is needed to wash away microorganisms from your hands.

• Use a common towel for you and others. Instead, use paper towels if possible. If not, use a separate clean towel for each person.

• Wear long or artificial (fake) nails when caring for someone. They promote the growth of pathogens.

• Wear a lot of jewellery because pathogens can grow well on them.

HANDWASHING REMINDERS

DO:

• Use a hand lotion (moisturizer) to prevent your hands from becoming dry and cracked. Dry, cracked or broken skin on the hands can make it easier for pathogens to enter and cause infections.

• Follow the rules of infection control. It is important to know when you should wash your hands and how to wash them correctly.

• Teach the people in your care and their families how and when to wash their hands.

Become a good role model.

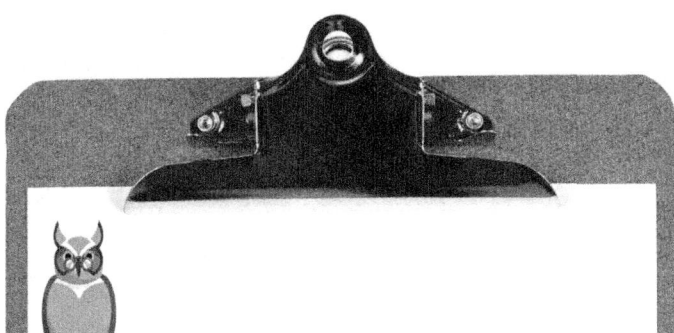

CHECK YOUR KNOWLEDGE

1. What are microorganisms?

2. What is a pathogen?

3. What 5 things are needed for the growth of microorganisms?

4. What 6 things are needed for an infection to occur?

5. What are the steps in the handwashing procedure?

6. When would you use a hand cleansing gel?

TEST YOURSELF

Please circle to indicate the best answer:

1. Most microorganisms are harmless and some even prevent us from getting sick.

a) True

b) False

2. Our body temperature is ideal for the growth of many microorganisms.

a) True

b) False

3. A mode of transmission is:

a) The way for a pathogen to be spread.

b) A source for the pathogen.

c) A way for the pathogen to enter a host.

4. Which of the following are steps in the handwashing procedure?

a) Keep fingernails short.

b) Use plenty of lather and friction for 10 to 15 seconds.

c) Use a nailbrush to scrub under the nails.

d) A and C

e) All of the above

5. You should wash your hands after removing your gloves.

a) True

b) False

6. While washing your hands, you should use a paper towel to turn the faucet on and off.

a) True

b) False

7. Hand cleansing gels can be used at all times to totally replace soap and water.

a) True

b) False

ANSWERS:

1. a) True. Many microorganisms are actually helpful to humans and help us to survive.

2. a) True. Our body temperature promotes the growth of many microorganisms.

3. a) A mode of transmission is a phrase that denotes how a pathogen spreads.

4. e) If you need to, refer to your notes and you'll see that all of these answers are correct.

5. a) True. This should be done as a precautionary measure.

6. a) True. This will ensure that you do not pick up pathogens from the faucet.

7. b) False. These gels should not replace soap and water. Even though they kill many pathogens, they do not remove dirt and soil. They can be used at times when it is hard to get to a sink.

REFERENCES

Breuninger, C., Follin, S., Munden, J., Munson, C., & Wittig, P. (Eds.). (2001). Handbook of nursing procedures. Pennsylvania: Springhouse.

Earl, M.L., Jackson, M.M., & Rickman, L. S. (2001). Improved rates of compliance with hand antisepsis guidelines: A three phase observational study. American Journal of Nursing, 101 (3), 26-33.

Garner, J. S. & Hospital Infection Control Advisory Committee (1996). Guidelines for isolation precautions in hospitals. American Journal of Infection Control, 24-52.

Health Canada. (1998). Infection control guidelines: Handwashing, cleaning and sterilization in healthcare. Ottawa.

Health Canada. (1997). Preventing the transmission of bloodborne pathogens in healthcare and public service settings. Canada Communicable Disease Report. Ottawa: Health Canada.

Hudek, K. (2001). Come on nurses: Wash your hands. Canadian Nurse, 97(9), 31-32.

Larson, L., & APIC Guideline Committee. (1995). Guidelines for handwashing and hand antisepsis in health care settings. American Journal of infection control, 23, 251-69.

Maggio, M. (1998). Quotations for a man's soul. Paramus, NJ: Prentice Hall.

Potter, P. A., & Perry, A. G. (2001). Canadian fundamentals of nursing. St. Louis: Mosby.

Smith, F.S., Duell, D.J., & Martin, B. C. (2000). Clinical nursing skills: Basic to advanced. (5th ed.). Toronto: Prentice Hall.

Walling, A. D. (2001). Hand hygiene during routine patient care is important. American Family Physician. [Onine]. Retrieved November 8th, 2001 from the world wide web. http://www,findarticles.com/cf_dm3225/8_63/74268416/print.jhtml.

Whiller, J., & Cooper, T. (2000). Clean hands: How to encourage good hygiene by patients. Nursing times, 94 (46), 37-38.

Zucker, E. (2000). Being a homemaker/home health aide. (5th ed.). Toronto: Prentice Hall.

Printed in Great Britain
by Amazon

59075226R00030